HOT DOGS
Hot Dogs
HOT DOGS
HOT DOGS

HotDogs Anonymous

by Sarah Bridges

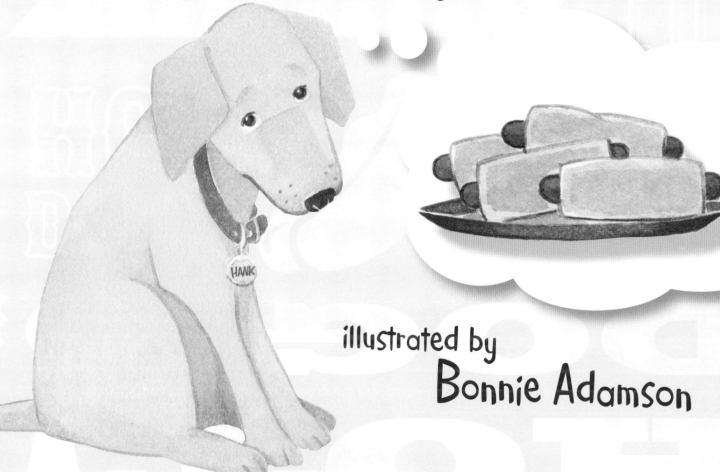

illustrated by
Bonnie Adamson

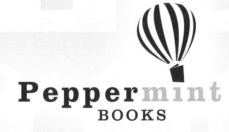

Peppermint
BOOKS

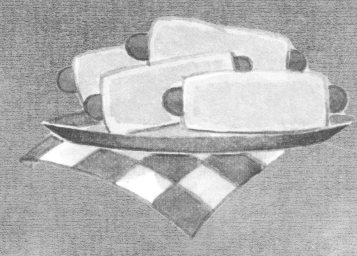

For anyone who's ever had a problem
they couldn't solve alone

For additional copies, visit www.sarahbridges.com

PUBLISHED BY:
Peppermint Books
P.O. Box 16512
Minneapolis, MN 55416
Visit Peppermint Books at
www.peppermintbooks.com

Publisher: Terri Foley
Copyeditor: Sandy Whelan
Art Director: Keith Griffin, Blue Tricycle, Inc.
Designer & Page Production: Heather Griffin, Blue Tricycle, Inc.

Publisher's Cataloging-in-Publication Data
(Provided by Quality Books, Inc.)
Bridges, Sarah.
  Hotdogs Anonymous / by Sarah Bridges ; illustrator,
  Bonnie Adamson
       p. cm.
SUMMARY: Hank, a yellow lab, is addicted to hot dogs.
His neighborhood dog pals convince him to go to a
Hotdogs Anonymous meeting. He finds support and
encouragement there. Through the help of the meeting, he
is on the road to recovery.
LCCN 2010936546
ISBN-13: 978-0-9828852-0-8
ISBN-10: 0-9828852-0-2
1. Frankfurters--Juvenile fiction. 2. Labrador
retriever--Juvenile fiction. 3. Compulsive eaters--
Juvenile fiction. 4. Twelve-step programs--Juvenile
fiction. [1. Frankfurters--Fiction. 2. Labrador
retriever--Fiction. 3. Compulsive eaters--Fiction.
4. Twelve-step programs--Fiction.] I. Adamson, Bonnie, ill.
II. Title.

PZ7.B7614Hot 2010   [E]
       QBI10-600190

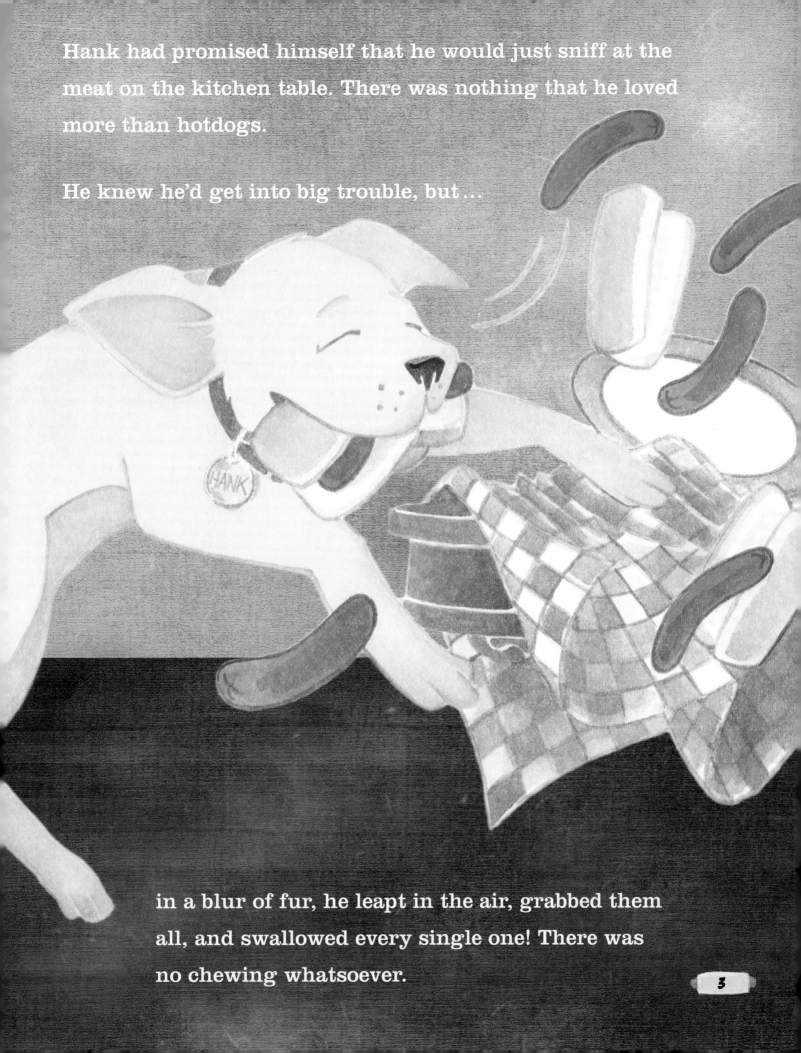

Hank had promised himself that he would just sniff at the meat on the kitchen table. There was nothing that he loved more than hotdogs.

He knew he'd get into big trouble, but...

in a blur of fur, he leapt in the air, grabbed them all, and swallowed every single one! There was no chewing whatsoever.

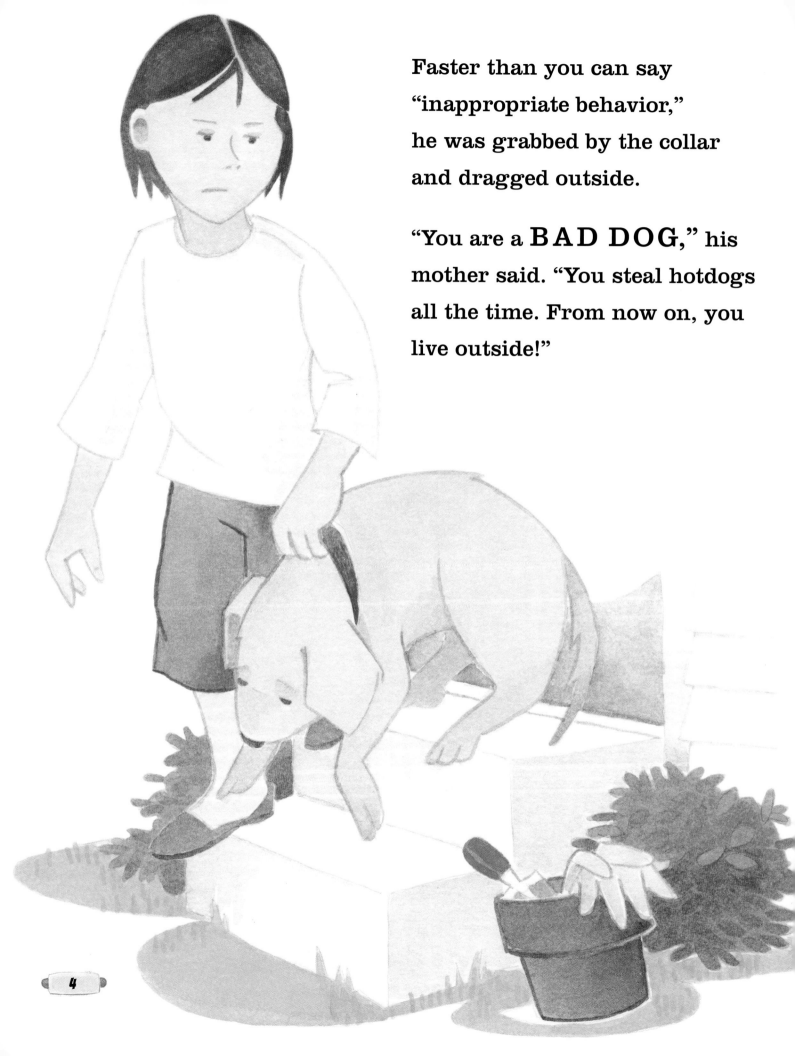

Faster than you can say "inappropriate behavior," he was grabbed by the collar and dragged outside.

"You are a **BAD DOG**," his mother said. "You steal hotdogs all the time. From now on, you live outside!"

"He didn't mean to, Mom,"
said Jackson.

"He must have missed
breakfast," echoed Noah.

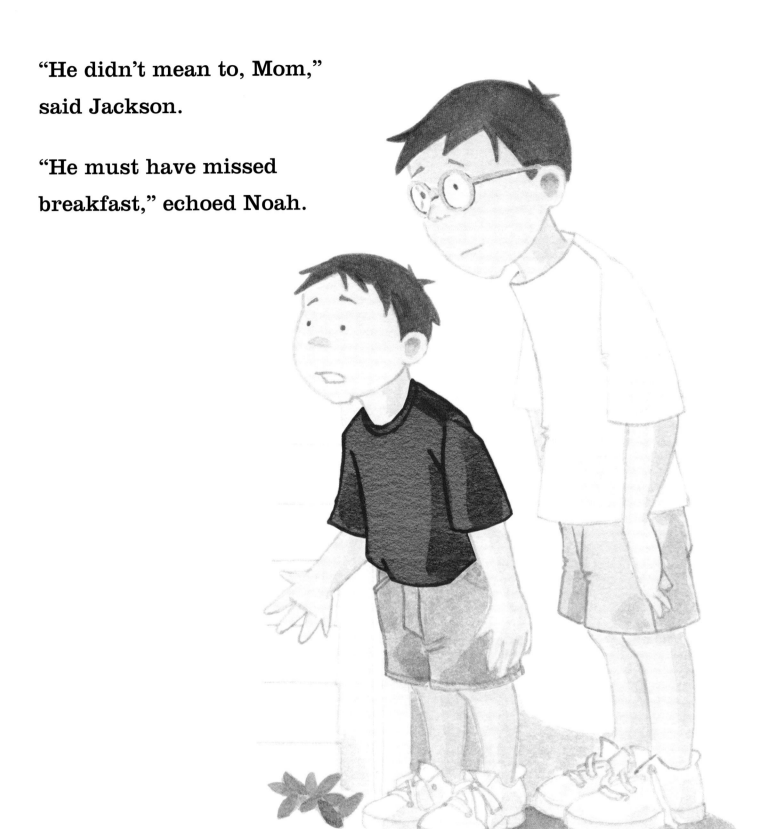

But Hank *had* meant to grab them and he *had* eaten
breakfast. He just *needed* those hotdogs.

Hank's stomach rumbled. Hotdogs had a way of talking back.

But he couldn't resist them.

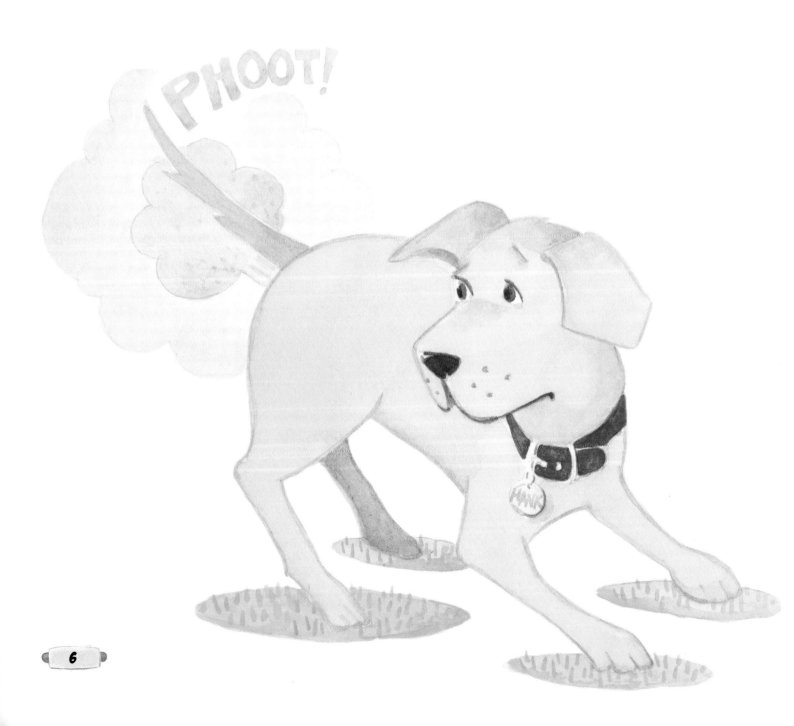

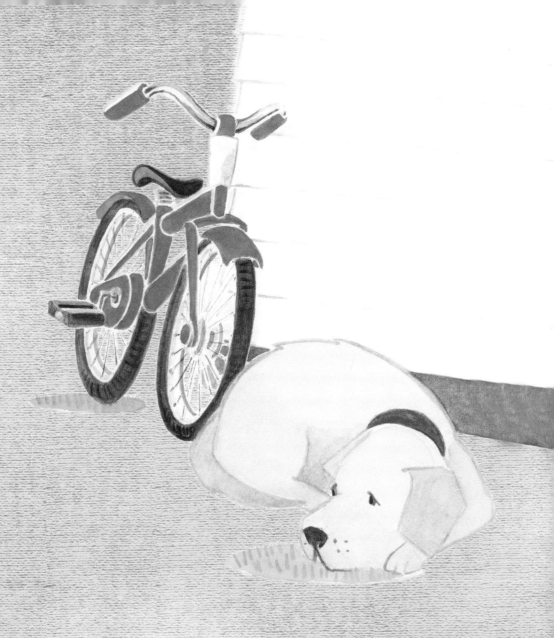

When his family went back inside, shame and remorse washed over Hank.

He knew he was in trouble. It was awful to have a problem and not know how to solve it. He vowed never to eat hotdogs again.

A day later, the neighborhood dogs arrived to help Hank kick his hotdog habit.

They were friends of Beagle W. and ready to intervene. They came from every breed and every type of family.

Each of them told *horrible, embarrassing* tales of Hank's hotdog-eating behavior.

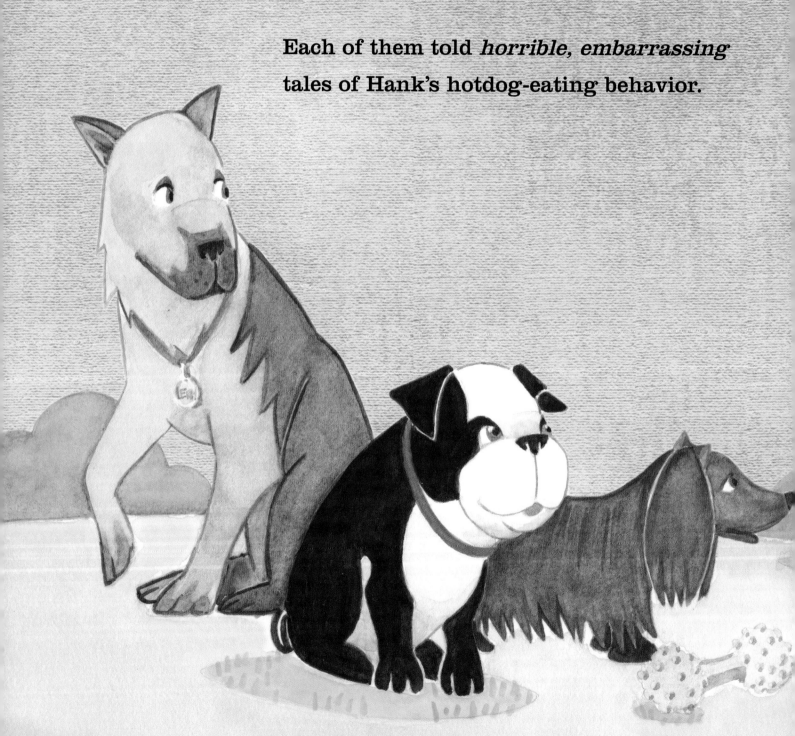

"I'll never forget when you came over to the barbeque at my two-legger's house and stole the plate of foot-long hotdogs," began Elsa, a well-groomed Dachshund. "I took the rap for that after you ran away."

"You did the same thing at my house," said Albert the Doberman, "wolfing down the leftover chili dogs and then complaining that you were sick, saying that you must have had one too many."

"It was cheese dogs, not chili dogs," Hank said lamely.
"I only had one!"

Hank tried to act natural. He tried to look innocent—small and
sweet, like a puppy. The other dogs didn't fall for it.

"You have a progressive condition, Hank," Louis said.

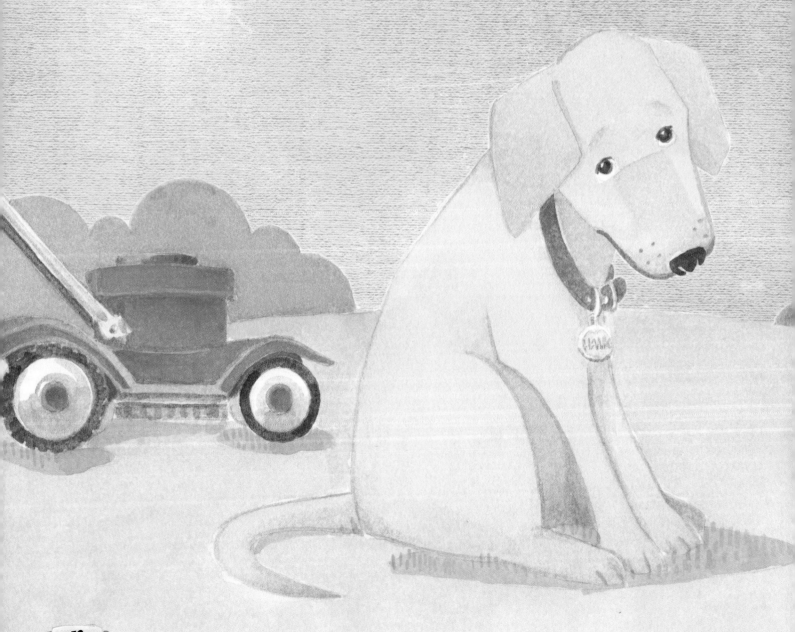

"You started like we all do—first sneaking a bite at a picnic, then eating out of the garbage, and finally, stealing from your own family!"

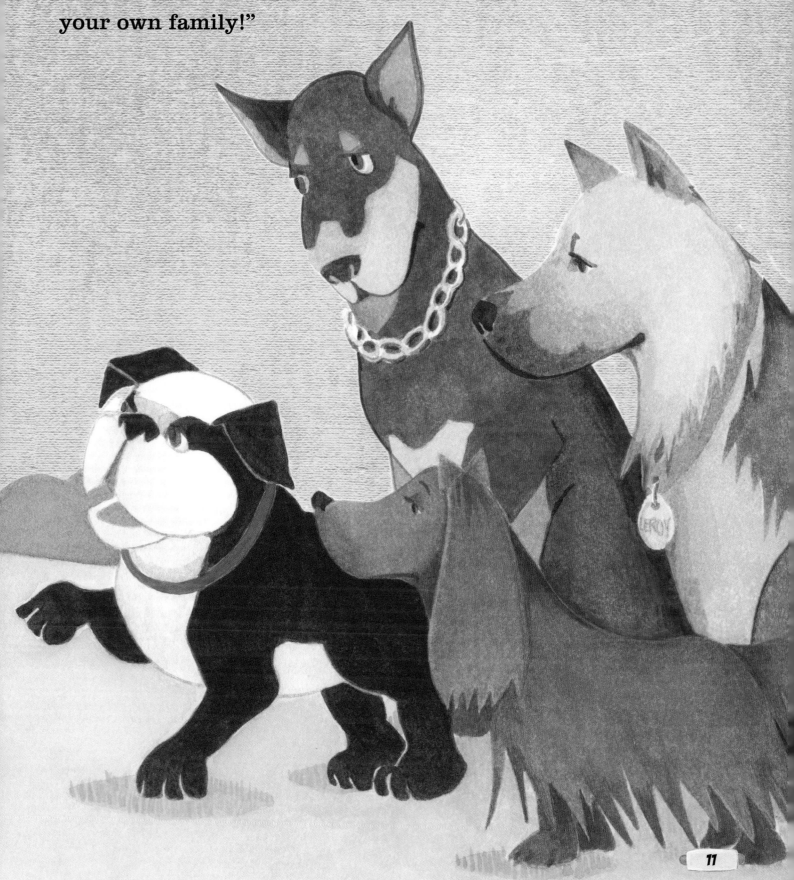

"But the hotdogs were cold," Hank whined. "Nobody even wanted them."

"That's your disease talking," Leroy barked. "You have a hotdog habit. Case closed."

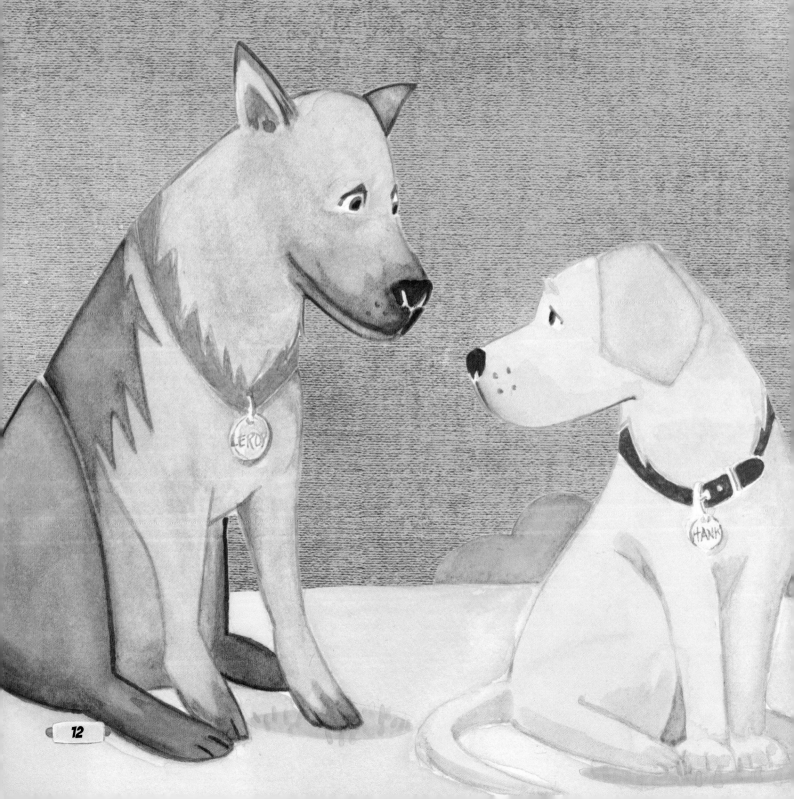

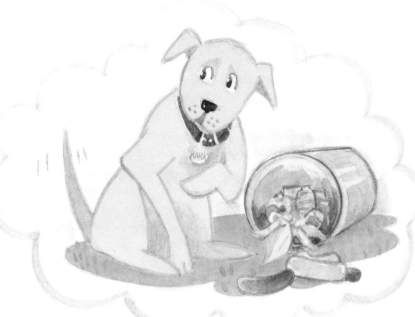

Hank hung his head. One hotdog was never enough. Once he got started, he couldn't stop.

He remembered the ruined holidays, the lies, and the friends who had written him off.

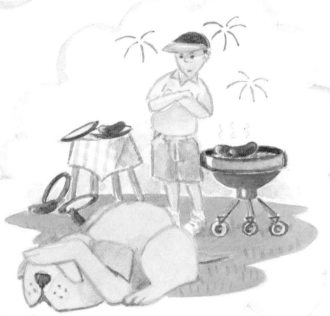

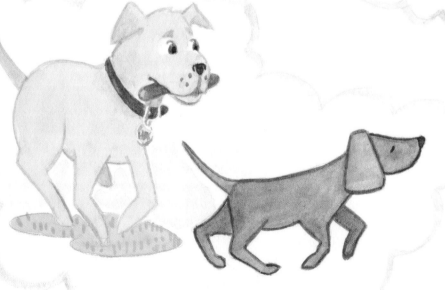

The neighborhood dogs were right. He had a hotdog habit.

"I've tried to quit before," Hank pleaded.

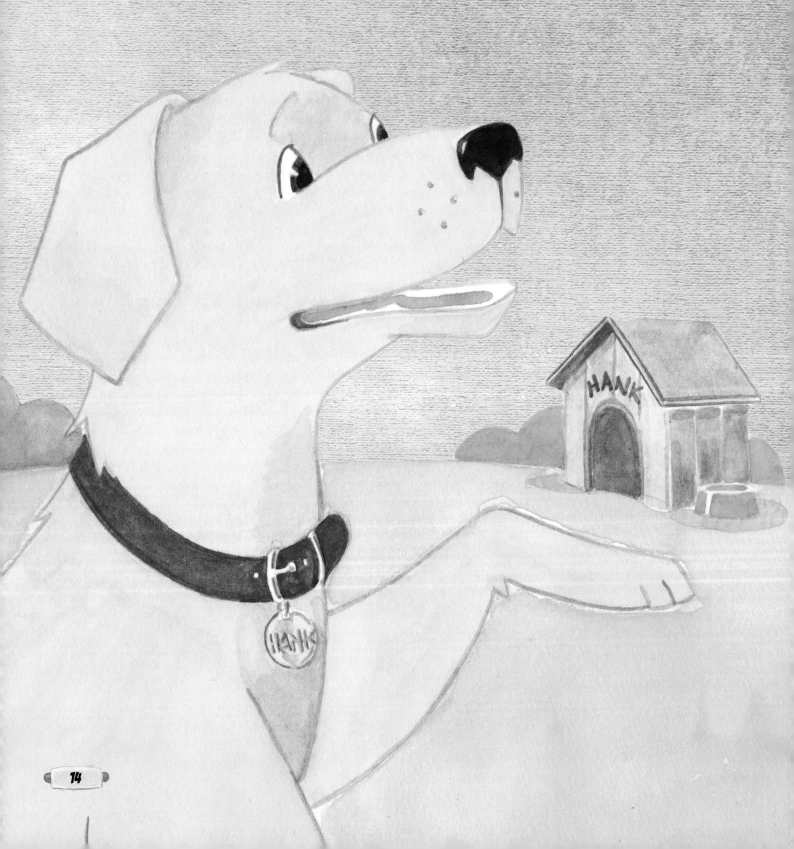

He had tried
hotdog-flavored
kibble.

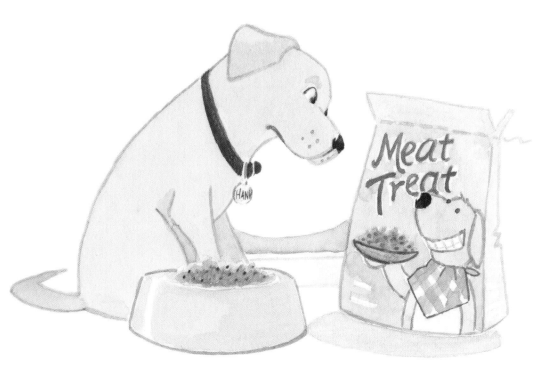

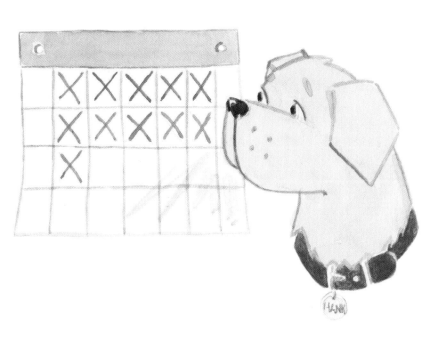

He had tried eating
hotdogs only
on weekends.

He had tried tofu dogs.
Nothing worked.

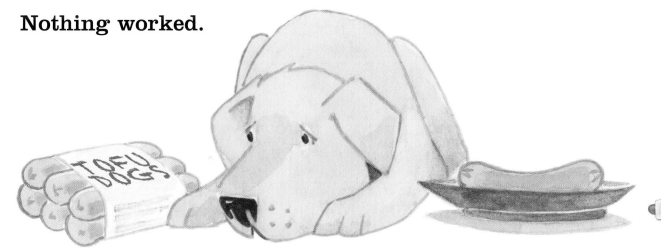

Two days later, Hank went to his first meeting of Hotdogs Anonymous.

It was held in a church basement: bad coffee, folding chairs, and slogans on the wall to boost their spirits.

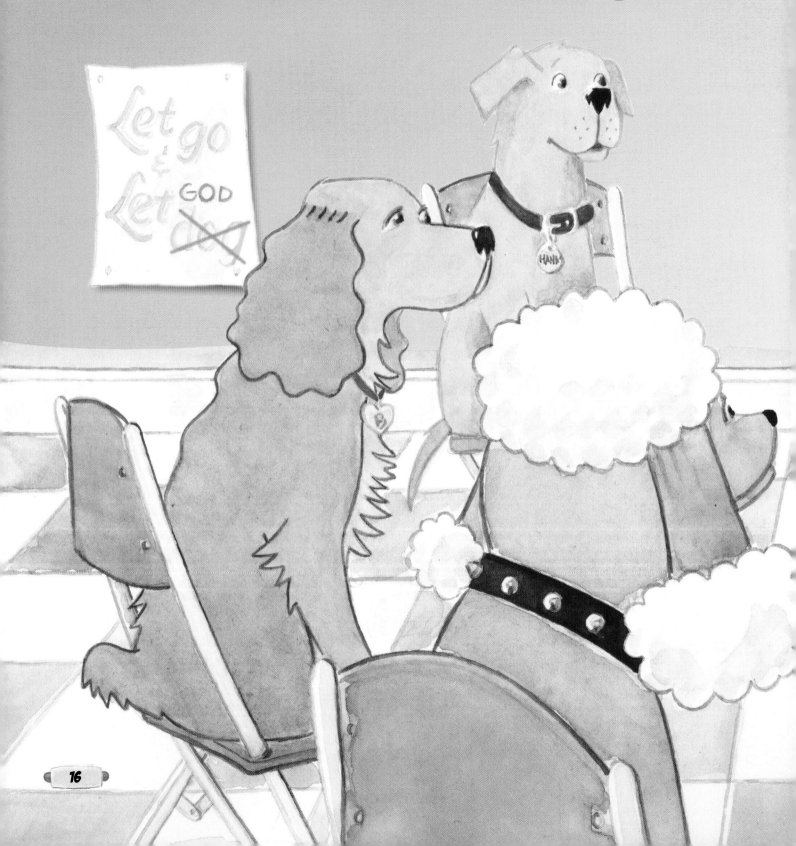

They sat in a circle. A Basset Hound went first. "I'm Bingo, and I have a hotdog habit."

The group responded in unison, "Hi, Bingo."

"My hotdog of choice is Vienna sausages—I love those little devils."

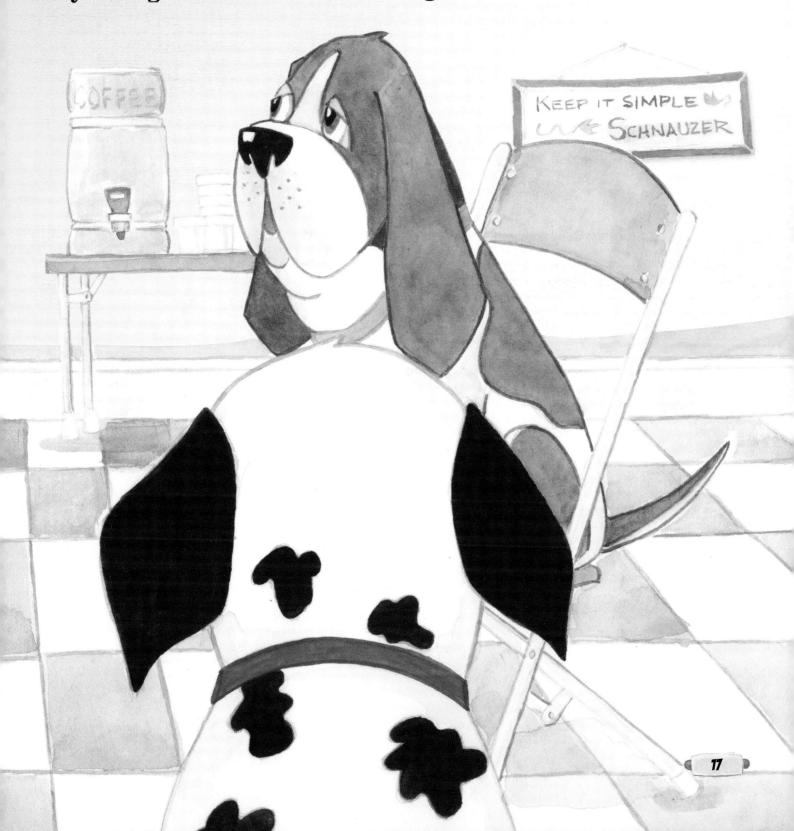

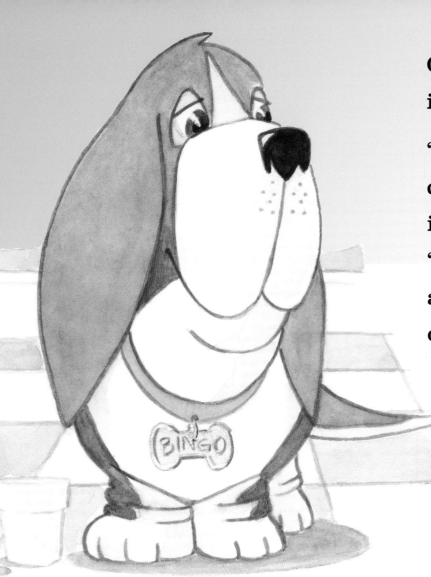

One by one the dogs introduced themselves.

"Because you're a new-comer, I'll tell you how it works," Bingo said. "The first step is to admit you're powerless over hotdogs."

The dogs nodded. Someone in the back growled.

Hank felt out of sorts. There was no way he was as bad as the other dogs.

Just a minute ago, a corndog-loving Miniature Poodle named Thunder had told a whopper of a hotdog-a-logue.

"I started with half a corndog and next thing I knew I was at the Minneapolis Zoo chasing a 200-pound pig ... and I'm a kosher dog."

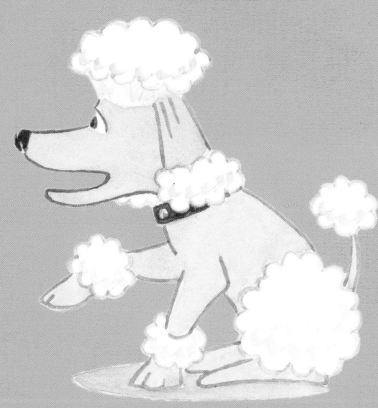

It got worse from there. Thunder continued, "After eating jumbo hotdogs until midnight, I woke up three states over married to a Timber Wolf—and they eat small dogs!"

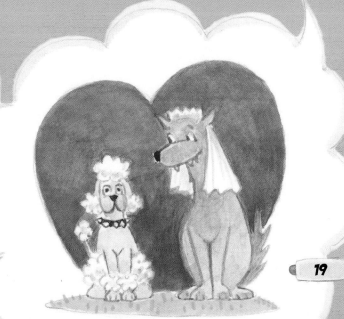

As much as Hank wanted to deny it, he knew he was one of them—he was a hotdog hound.

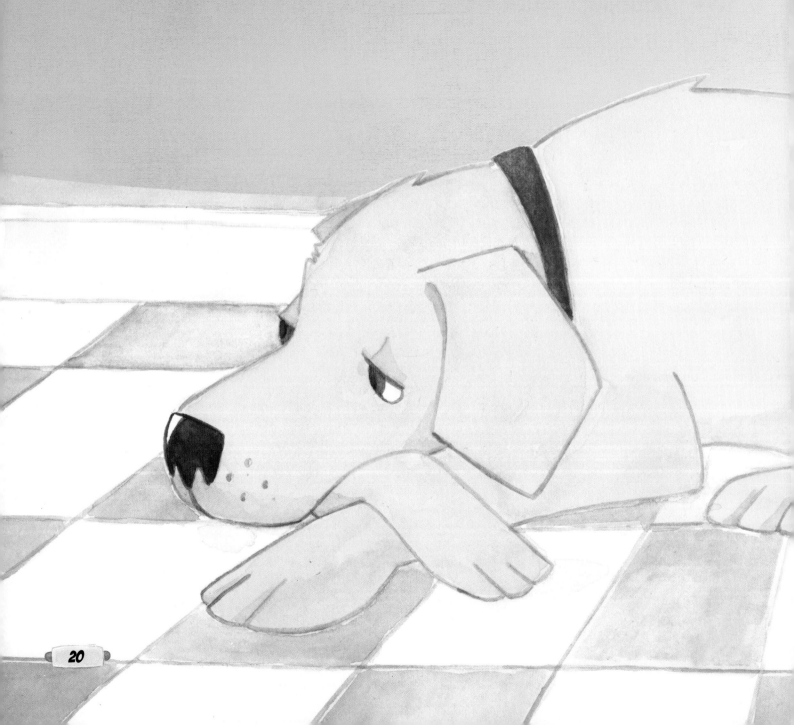

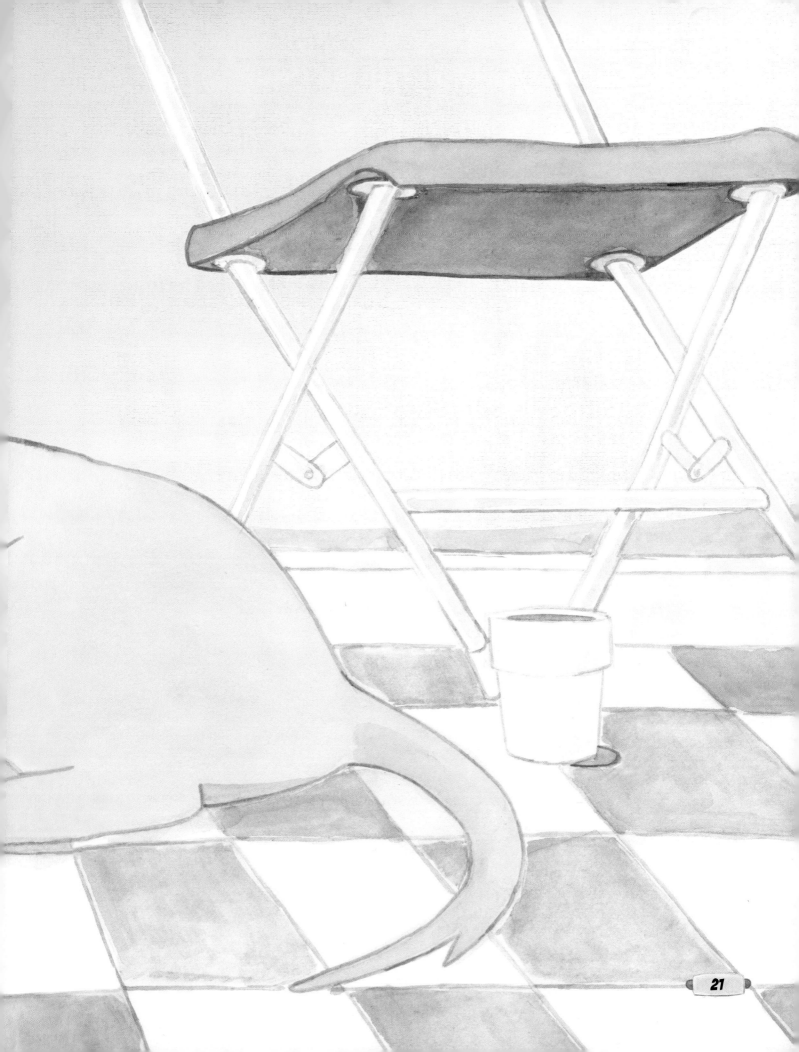

"Tell us your story, Hank," said a Dalmatian named Rover.

Hank began reluctantly. "Several years ago, I got caught hiding hotdogs around the house. My owners said they attracted mice."

There were knowing looks in the group.

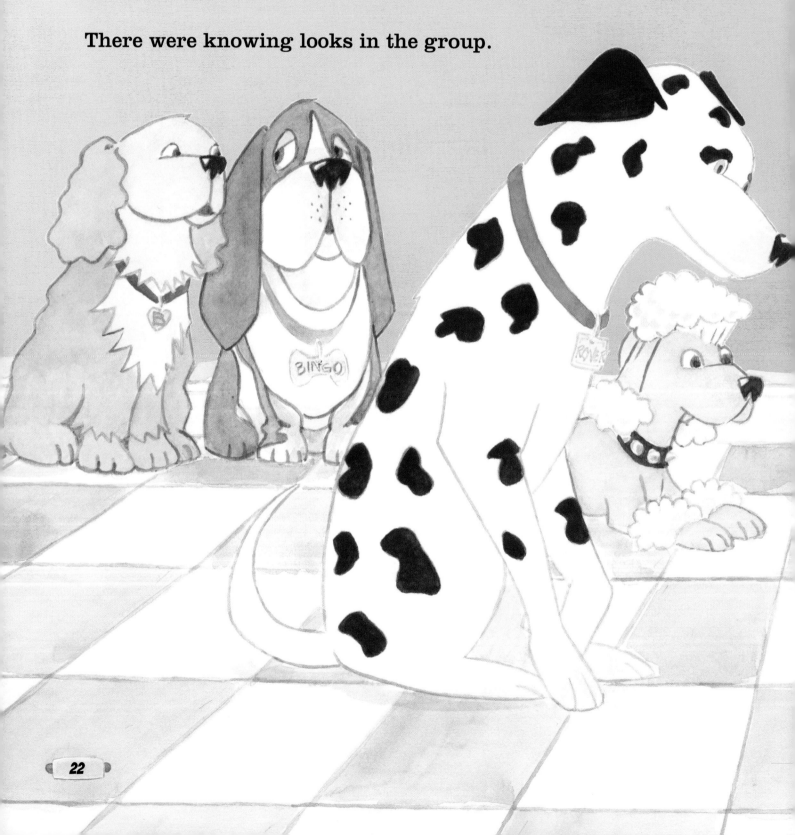

Hank told about when he had tried switching from hotdogs to other meats—something Thunder called the *chicken experiment*.

As he told his stories, he felt better because he could tell that these folks knew what he was talking about ... some even had worse stories than his.

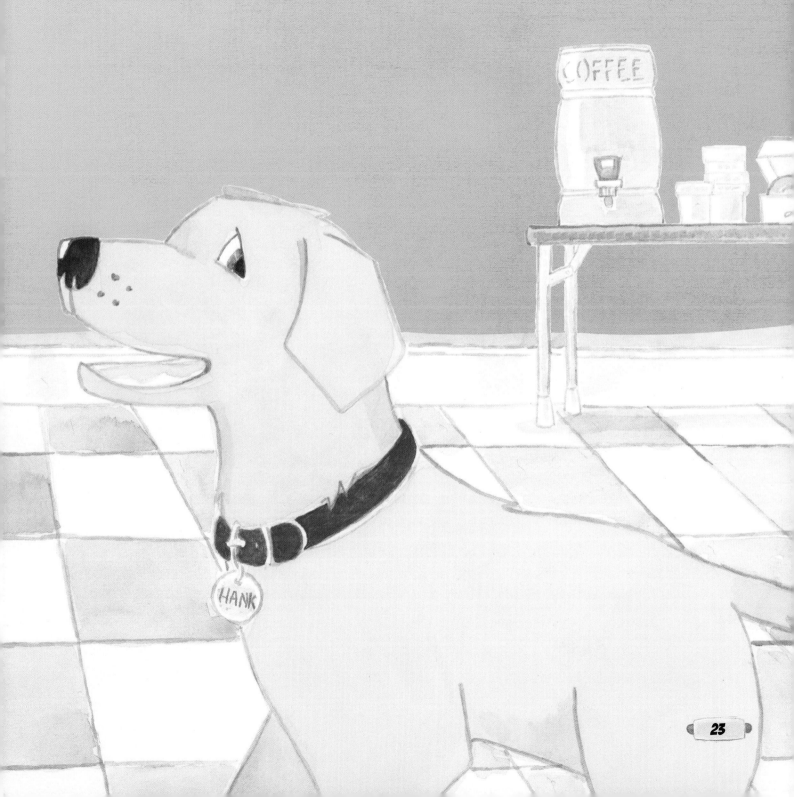

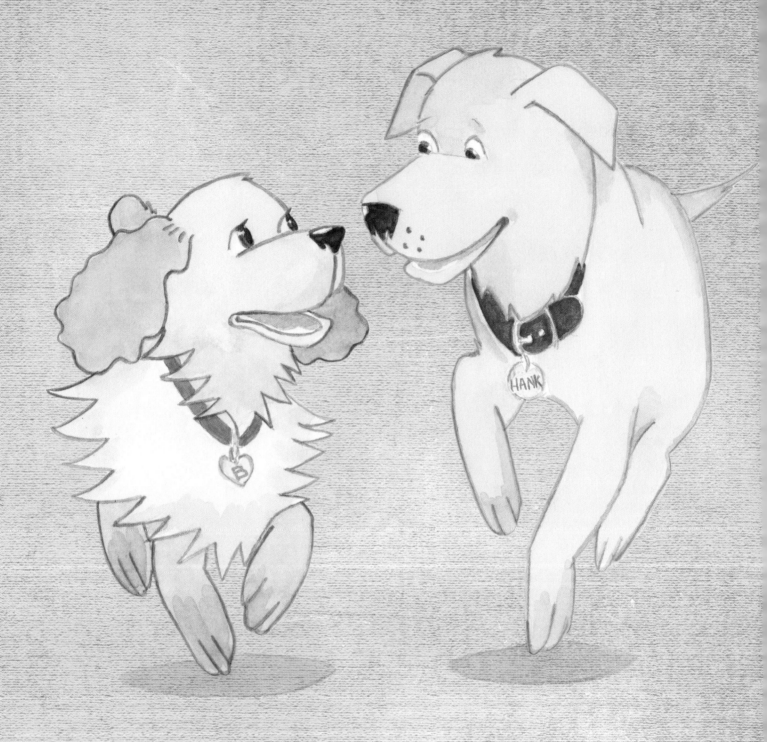

Hank left the meeting feeling relieved and even happy.
He wasn't alone anymore with his habit. He had some help.

"Easy Dog It," said Billi as they sniffed each other and
said good-bye.

He felt like he was
floating on a pink cloud.

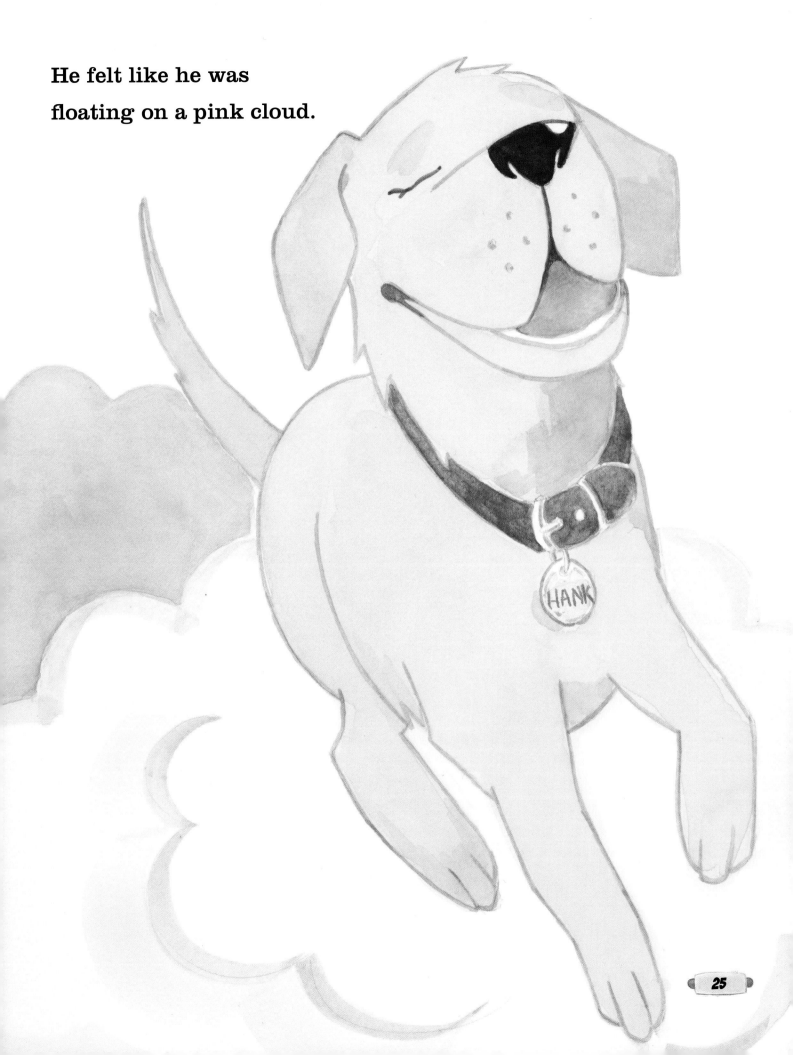

Hank began practicing what
he'd learned in the meeting.

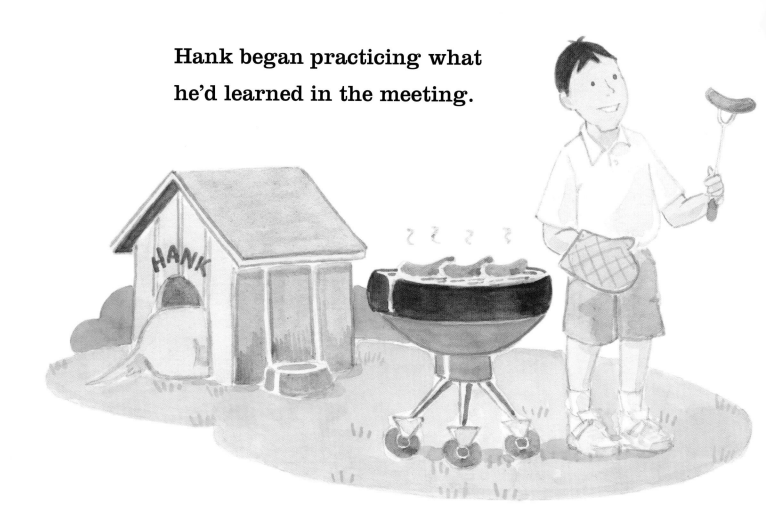

He avoided the first hotdog and barked for help when he
felt a hotdog urge. His friends came running.

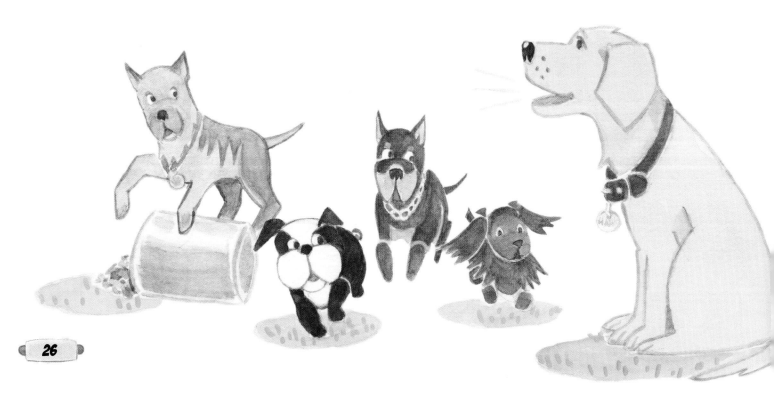

Within weeks the change was astounding. At the next meeting, Thunder said, "You look like a million bones!"

Hank was working hard on improving himself and on becoming less resentful of other dogs—the normal ones who could have one hotdog and then stop.

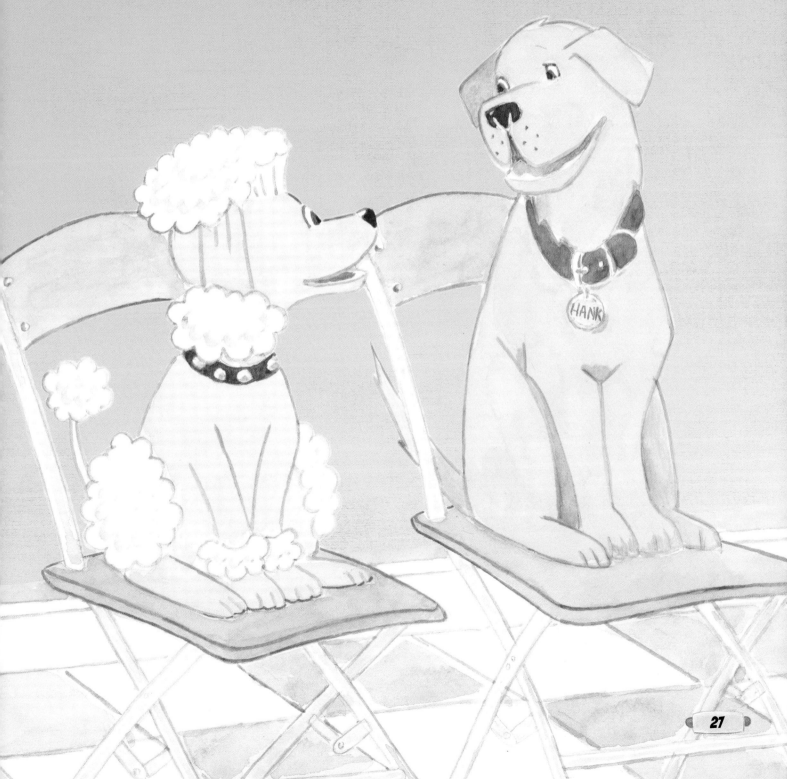

A few months
later, his family
allowed him back
into the house.

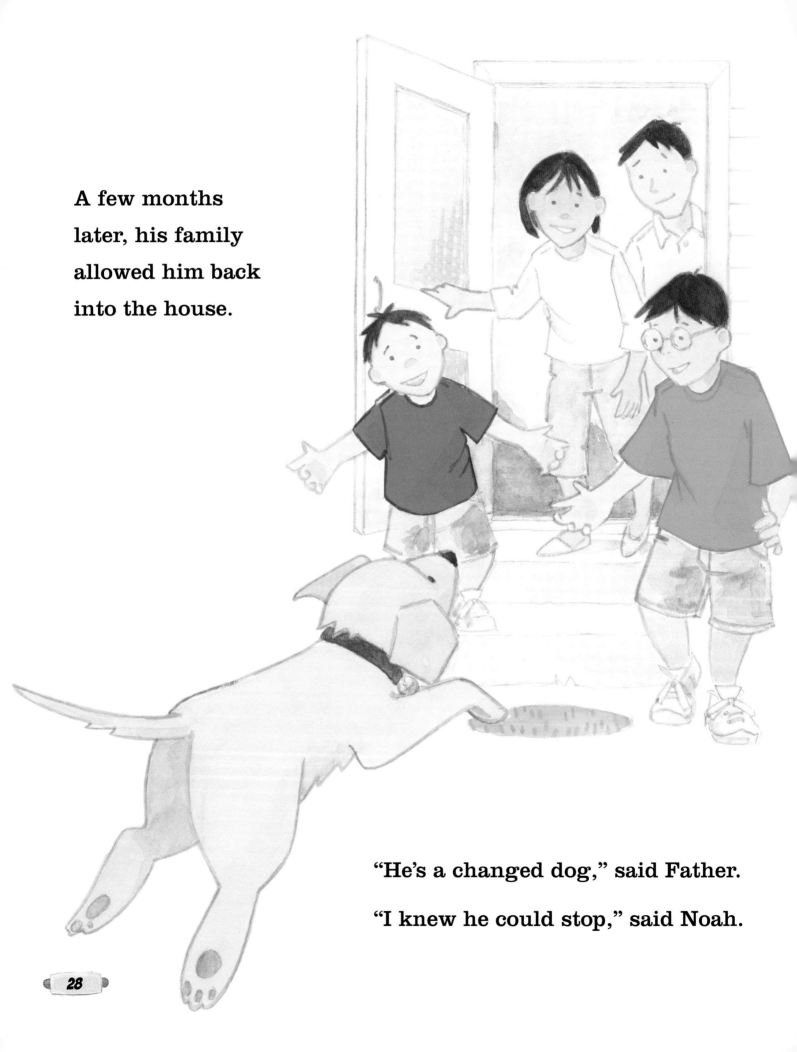

"He's a changed dog," said Father.

"I knew he could stop," said Noah.

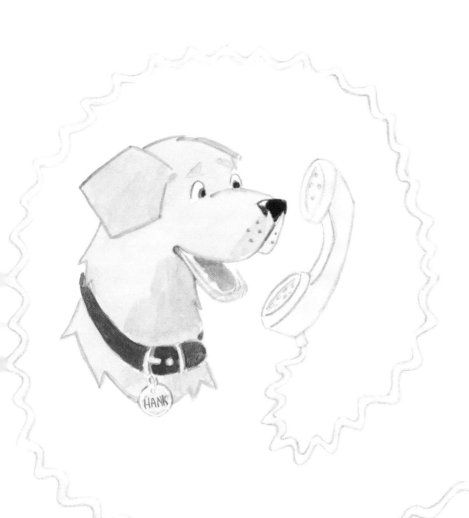

It wasn't all easy,
but Hank loved the
feeling of confronting
his hotdog problem.

When he got the craving
for hotdogs, he'd call
Thunder for reassurance.

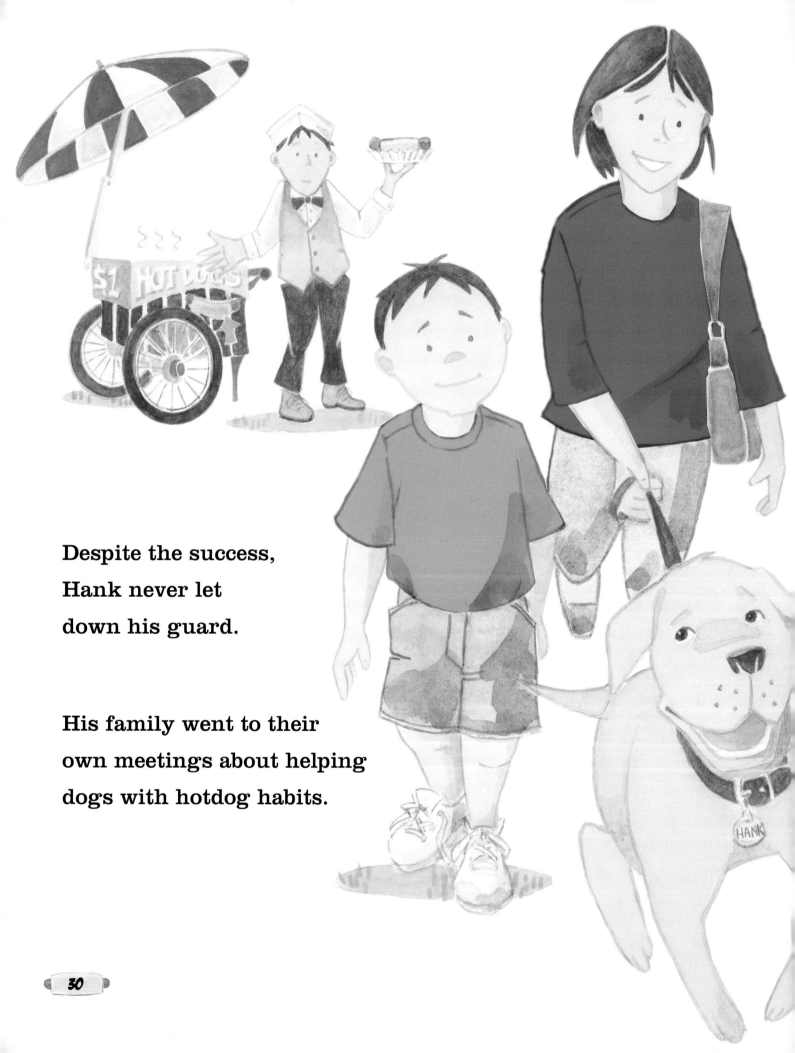

Despite the success,
Hank never let
down his guard.

His family went to their
own meetings about helping
dogs with hotdog habits.

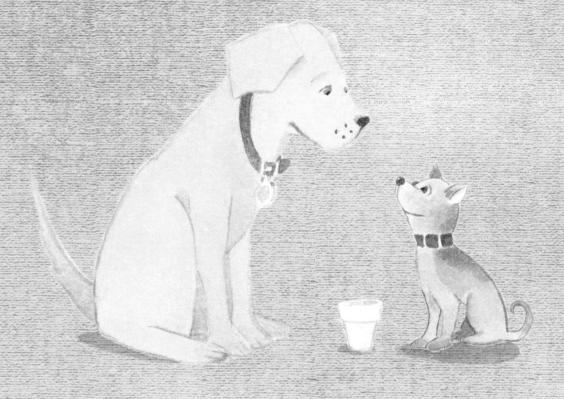

Hank was on the road to recovery.

As he told a newcomer at his meeting one night, "Remember, we deal with hotdogs ... cunning, baffling, powerful!"

His advice was to just take it one day at a time.

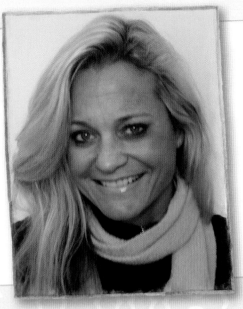

AUTHOR :: Sarah Bridges, PhD

Sarah Bridges, PhD, is a psychologist and writer living in Minneapolis with her four children. She has written 13 children's books including Hank's story. She grew up in a commune in California where she first became interested in personal growth and psychology. In the rest of her life, she works with business people to help them become better leaders. She loves to read, run, and watch her kids play sports.

ILLUSTRATOR :: Bonnie Adamson

Bonnie is a freelance print designer as well as an illustrator of children's books. She and her obsessively supportive husband live in South Carolina with two grown daughters close by. Bonnie loves to spoil her grand-dogs, Andy and Mabel, with bacon treats and hotdogs whenever possible.

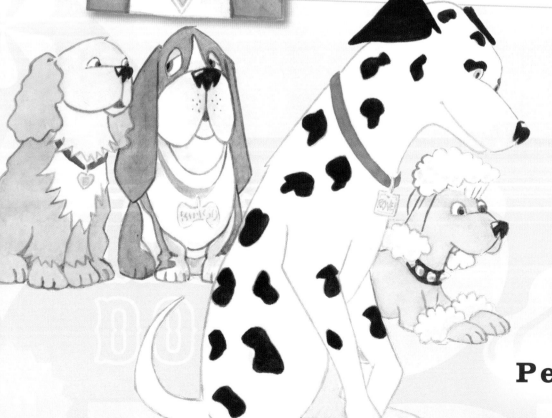

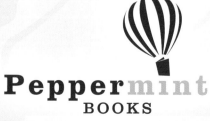

Peppermint
BOOKS